FULL LIQUID DIET

Nutritious Meal Replacement
for Health & Weight Loss

Roger R. Hackett

CONTENTS

Title Page

Copyright

Preface

CHAPTER ONE   1

CHAPTER TWO   16

CHAPTER FOUR   23

CHAPTER FIVE   29

CHAPTER SIX   34

CHAPTER SEVEN   40

CHAPTER EIGHT   46

CONCLUSION   75

PREFACE

Dear Reader,

Thank you for choosing this book on the Full Liquid Diet. This diet is often recommended for individuals who have difficulty chewing, swallowing, or digesting solid foods, and is often used in medical settings before or after surgeries or procedures.

In this book, I have compiled a comprehensive guide on the Full Liquid Diet, including what it is, who it's for, and how to follow it safely and effectively. I have also included a variety of recipes and meal plans to help you navigate this diet and ensure that you are getting all the nutrients you need.

As a registered dietitian and nutritionist, I have seen firsthand the benefits of this diet for individuals with various medical conditions. However, it is important to note that this diet is not appropriate for everyone and should only be followed under the guidance of a healthcare provider.

I hope that this book provides you with the knowledge and resources you need to successfully follow the Full Liquid Diet and improve your overall health and well-being.

CHAPTER ONE

INTRODUCTION

Definition Of Full Liquid Diet

A full liquid diet is a type of diet that consists of foods that are liquid or can be turned into liquid form at room temperature. This type of diet is prescribed for individuals who are unable to consume solid foods due to medical conditions or surgeries. Full liquid diets typically exclude solid foods, as well as any food that requires chewing, such as fruits, vegetables, and meats. Instead, these diets include foods such as milk, yogurt, fruit juices, broths, and certain types of pudding or gelatin.

Full liquid diets can be used as a short-term measure to help individuals recover from a medical condition or surgery. They can also be used as a long-term dietary strategy for individuals who have difficulty chewing or swallowing solid foods due to conditions such as dysphagia or certain types of cancer.

Why Is Full Liquid Diet Prescribed?

Full liquid diets are often prescribed for a variety of medical reasons. They may be recommended for individuals who are recovering from surgery or who have medical conditions that make it difficult to chew or swallow solid foods. Some common reasons for prescribing a full liquid diet include:

1. After surgery: After certain types of surgery, such as gastrointestinal surgery, it may be necessary to follow a full liquid diet for a period of time to allow the body to heal and recover.

2. Medical conditions: Individuals with medical conditions such as dysphagia, Crohn's disease, or certain types of cancer may find it difficult or uncomfortable to eat solid foods. In these cases, a full liquid diet may be recommended as a long-term dietary strategy.

3. Dental procedures: After certain dental

procedures, such as tooth extraction or oral surgery, it may be necessary to follow a full liquid diet for a period of time to allow the mouth to heal.

4. Weight loss: Some individuals may choose to follow a full liquid diet as a short-term strategy for weight loss. However, it is important to note that this type of diet is not recommended for long-term weight loss or for individuals who have a history of disordered eating.

Types Of Full Liquid Diet

There are several different types of full liquid diets, each with its own specific guidelines and restrictions. Some common types of full liquid diets include:

1. Clear liquid diet: This type of diet consists of clear liquids such as water, broth, clear fruit juices, and certain types of sports drinks. Solid foods and milk products are not allowed on a clear liquid diet.

2. Full liquid diet: A full liquid diet consists of foods that are liquid at room temperature, as well as foods that can be blended or pureed into a liquid form. This may include foods such as milk, yogurt, fruit juices, broths, and certain types of pudding or gelatin.

3. Pureed diet: A pureed diet consists of foods that have been pureed or blended to a smooth consistency. This may include foods such as soups, vegetables, and meats.

4. Mechanical soft diet: A mechanical soft diet consists of foods that are soft and easy to chew, such as ground meats, cooked vegetables, and soft fruits.

It is important to note that full liquid diets should only be followed under the guidance of a healthcare professional. In some cases, it may be necessary to supplement the diet with vitamins and minerals to ensure that the individual is receiving adequate nutrition.

Benefits Of Full Liquid Diet

Full liquid diets can provide a variety of benefits for individuals who are unable to consume solid foods. Some potential benefits of a full liquid diet include:

1. Improved hydration: Liquid diets can help individuals maintain proper hydration levels, which is important for overall health and wellbeing.

2. Reduced stress on the digestive system: Liquid diets can help reduce stress on the digestive

system, which may be beneficial for individuals recovering from surgery.

3. Easier to digest: Liquid diets can be easier for the body to digest, which can be beneficial for individuals with certain medical conditions or who have undergone surgery.

4. Can be nutritionally balanced: A full liquid diet can be designed to be nutritionally balanced, with a variety of liquids and pureed foods that provide the necessary vitamins, minerals, and other nutrients.

5. Can help with weight loss: While not recommended as a long-term weight loss strategy, a full liquid diet can help individuals lose weight in the short-term by reducing overall caloric intake.

It is important to note that full liquid diets should only be followed under the guidance of a healthcare professional, as they may not be appropriate for everyone. Individuals who follow a full liquid diet for an extended period of time may be at risk for malnutrition and other health issues if the diet is not properly balanced.

In addition, some individuals may experience side effects such as nausea, diarrhea, or constipation when following a full liquid diet. It is important to monitor these symptoms and make adjustments to the diet as necessary.

Overall, while a full liquid diet may not be the most enjoyable or satisfying way to eat, it can provide important benefits for individuals who are unable to consume solid foods. By working closely with a healthcare professional, individuals can ensure that their full liquid diet is nutritionally balanced and appropriate for their unique needs and medical conditions.

What You Can And Cannot Eat On A Full Liquid Diet

List of Allowed Foods

When following a specific diet, it is essential to know the list of allowed foods to ensure that you are eating the right things. Some diets may restrict certain types of foods, while others may allow them in moderation. Here is a list of allowed foods that you can incorporate into your diet.

Fruits and Vegetables

Fruits and vegetables are essential components of a healthy diet. They provide vital nutrients and fiber that are necessary for good health. The following fruits and vegetables are allowed on most diets:

- Apples, bananas, berries, citrus fruits, and other low-sugar fruits

- Leafy greens, such as spinach, kale, and collard greens

- Cruciferous vegetables, such as broccoli, cauliflower, and Brussels sprouts

- Root vegetables, such as sweet potatoes, carrots, and beets

- Other vegetables, such as cucumbers, bell peppers, and tomatoes

Protein Sources

Protein is essential for building and repairing muscles, and it also plays a vital role in maintaining a healthy immune system. Here are some protein sources that are allowed on most diets:

- Lean meats, such as chicken, turkey, and fish

- Eggs and egg whites

- Low-fat dairy products, such as milk, yogurt, and cheese

- Plant-based protein sources, such as beans,

lentils, tofu, and tempeh

Grains and Starches

Grains and starches provide the body with energy and fiber. Here are some grains and starches that are allowed on most diets:

- Whole grains, such as brown rice, quinoa, and whole-grain bread
- Starchy vegetables, such as potatoes and corn
- Legumes, such as lentils and beans

Fats and Oils

Fats and oils are essential for good health, but they should be consumed in moderation. Here are some fats and oils that are allowed on most diets:

- Olive oil, coconut oil, and other plant-based oils
- Nuts and seeds, such as almonds, walnuts, chia seeds, and flaxseeds
- Avocadoes

Other Foods

Here are some other foods that are allowed on most diets:

- Herbs and spices

- Unsweetened beverages, such as water, tea, and coffee
- Low-sugar condiments, such as mustard and salsa

It is essential to note that the list of allowed foods may vary depending on the specific diet you are following. It is important to consult with a registered dietitian or a healthcare professional before making any significant changes to your diet.

List of Prohibited Foods

In contrast to the list of allowed foods, there are also prohibited foods that should be avoided when following a specific diet. These foods may be high in calories, sugar, or fat, and they may not provide the necessary nutrients that the body needs. Here is a list of prohibited foods that you should avoid.

Processed Foods

Processed foods are often high in sugar, salt, and unhealthy fats. They may also contain additives and preservatives that can be harmful to the body. Here are some processed foods that should be avoided:

- Chips and other salty snacks
- Candy, chocolate, and other sweets
- Soda and other sugary beverages
- Fast food, such as burgers, fries, and pizza

High-Fat Foods

High-fat foods may be delicious, but they can also be harmful to the body. They are often high in calories and can lead to weight gain and other health problems. Here are some high-fat foods that should be avoided:

- Fried foods, such as fried chicken and French fries
- High-fat meats, such as bacon and sausage
- Full-fat dairy products, such as whole milk

Refined Carbohydrates

Refined carbohydrates are often stripped of their fiber and other nutrients, making them less healthy than their whole-grain counterparts. Here are some refined carbohydrates that should be avoided:

- White bread and other refined grains
- Pasta and other refined grain products
- Sugary breakfast cereals

High-Sugar Foods

High-sugar foods can cause blood sugar spikes and crashes, which can lead to a host of health problems. Here are some high-sugar foods that should be avoided:

- Candy, chocolate, and other sweets
- Sugary breakfast cereals
- Sugary drinks, such as soda and juice

Other Prohibited Foods

Here are some other foods that are generally prohibited on most diets:

- Alcohol and other sugary drinks
- Processed meats, such as hot dogs and deli meat
- High-sodium foods, such as canned soups and frozen meals

It is important to note that the list of prohibited foods may vary depending on the specific diet you are following. It is important to consult with a registered dietitian or a healthcare professional before making any significant changes to your diet.

Seven Days Sample Meal Plan For Full Liquid Diet

A full liquid diet is a type of diet that consists of liquids or foods that melt into liquids at room temperature. It is often used for medical purposes, such as after surgery or to treat digestive problems. Here is a sample seven-day meal plan for a full liquid diet.

Day One

- Breakfast: Protein shake made with whey protein powder, milk, and berries
- Snack: Clear broth
- Lunch: Cream of chicken soup made with chicken broth and heavy cream
- Snack: Sugar-free gelatin
- Dinner: Creamy tomato soup made with tomato juice and heavy cream

Day Two

- Breakfast: Smoothie made with milk, banana, and peanut butter
- Snack: Clear broth
- Lunch: Cream of broccoli soup made with

broccoli, chicken broth, and heavy cream

- Snack: Sugar-free pudding

- Dinner: Creamy cauliflower soup made with cauliflower, chicken broth, and heavy cream

Day Three

- Breakfast: Protein shake made with whey protein powder, milk, and strawberries

- Snack: Clear broth

- Lunch: Cream of mushroom soup made with mushrooms, chicken broth, and heavy cream

- Snack: Sugar-free gelatin

- Dinner: Creamy potato soup made with potatoes, chicken broth, and heavy cream

Day Four

- Breakfast: Smoothie made with milk, blueberries, and Greek yogurt

- Snack: Clear broth

- Lunch: Cream of asparagus soup made with asparagus, chicken broth, and heavy cream

- Snack: Sugar-free pudding

- Dinner: Creamy zucchini soup made with zucchini, chicken broth, and heavy cream

Day Five

- Breakfast: Protein shake made with whey

protein powder, milk, and raspberries

- Snack: Clear broth

- Lunch: Cream of celery soup made with celery, chicken broth, and heavy cream

- Snack: Sugar-free gelatin

- Dinner: Creamy pumpkin soup made with pumpkin puree, chicken broth, and heavy cream

Day Six

- Breakfast: Smoothie made with milk, peaches, and cottage cheese

- Snack: Clear broth

- Lunch: Cream of spinach soup made with spinach, chicken broth, and heavy cream

- Snack: Sugar-free pudding

- Dinner: Creamy butternut squash soup made with butternut squash, chicken broth, and heavy cream

Day Seven

- Breakfast: Protein shake made with whey protein powder, milk, and mixed berries

- Snack: Clear broth

- Lunch: Cream of tomato soup made with tomato juice and heavy cream

- Snack: Sugar-free gelatin

- Dinner: Creamy carrot soup made with carrots, chicken broth, and heavy cream

It is important to note that this meal plan is just an example and should not be followed without the guidance of a healthcare professional. A full liquid diet should only be followed for a short period of time and should not be used as a long-term dietary approach.

In addition, it is important to ensure that a full liquid diet provides adequate nutrients, such as protein and fiber. It may be necessary to supplement the diet with vitamins and minerals to avoid nutrient deficiencies.

CHAPTER TWO

Preparing for a Full Liquid Diet

Consultation With A Dietitian

Dietitians are trained professionals who can help individuals achieve and maintain a healthy diet. Consultation with a dietitian is essential for those who want to make significant changes to their dietary habits, such as those with chronic health conditions or those seeking to lose weight. A dietitian will work with an individual to develop a personalized diet plan that meets their specific needs.

What To Expect During A Consultation With A Dietitian?

During a consultation with a dietitian, an individual can

expect to discuss their current eating habits, health goals, and any medical conditions they may have. The dietitian will assess an individual's nutritional needs and create a plan that will help them achieve their goals. This plan may include specific foods to eat or avoid, portion control recommendations, and suggestions for supplements or alternative sources of nutrients.

The Benefits Of Consulting With A Dietitian

One of the benefits of consulting with a dietitian is that they can help an individual make sustainable changes to their eating habits. A dietitian can provide education on nutrition and help an individual understand the impact that their diet has on their overall health. A dietitian can also help an individual make choices that fit their lifestyle and preferences, making it easier for them to stick to their new diet plan.

Who Can Benefit From Consulting With A Dietitian?

Consulting with a dietitian can be beneficial for anyone looking to improve their health and wellbeing. This includes individuals with chronic conditions such as diabetes, high blood pressure, and heart disease. Those who are looking to lose weight or gain muscle can also benefit from consulting with a dietitian. Additionally, individuals who are pregnant or breastfeeding may need specific dietary recommendations to support their health and the health of their baby.

Shopping For Full Liquid Diet Foods

A full liquid diet is a type of diet that includes foods that are liquid or semi-solid at room temperature. This diet may be recommended for individuals who have difficulty chewing or swallowing, or those recovering from certain medical procedures. Shopping for full liquid diet foods can be challenging, as many foods that are typically considered staples are not suitable for this type of diet.

Foods To Include In A Full Liquid Diet

Foods that are suitable for a full liquid diet include broths, pureed soups, milk, and milk alternatives such as soy or almond milk. Yogurt, ice cream, and pudding are also acceptable as long as they are free of solid pieces. Juices, smoothies, and shakes are also good options, as are protein powders and liquid nutritional supplements.

Foods To Avoid In A Full Liquid Diet

Foods that are typically avoided in a full liquid diet include solid foods such as meats, vegetables, and fruits. This includes foods that are cooked but have a solid texture, such as oatmeal or mashed potatoes. Additionally, foods that are high in fiber, such as whole grains or raw vegetables, should be avoided as they can be difficult to digest.

Tips For Shopping For Full Liquid Diet Foods

When shopping for full liquid diet foods, it is important to read labels carefully and avoid any foods that contain solid pieces or are high in fiber. Look for products that are labeled as "pureed," "smooth," or "blended." It may also be helpful to stock up on broths, smoothie ingredients, and liquid

It may also be helpful to stock up on broths, smoothie ingredients, and liquid nutritional supplements to ensure that there are enough options available to meet nutritional needs.

It is also important to keep in mind that some full liquid diet foods may not be suitable for everyone. For example, individuals with lactose intolerance or allergies to certain foods may need to avoid milk-based products. It is recommended to consult with a dietitian or healthcare professional for personalized recommendations.

Kitchen Preparation And Equipment

When it comes to preparing meals, having the right kitchen equipment and preparation techniques can make a big difference. Whether an individual is cooking for themselves or for a group, having the right tools and knowledge can help make meal preparation faster, easier, and more enjoyable.

Essential Kitchen Equipment

Some essential kitchen equipment includes a sharp chef's knife, cutting board, pots and pans, mixing bowls, measuring cups and spoons, a blender, and a food processor. Other helpful tools include a vegetable peeler, a can opener, a garlic press, and a zester. It is also important to have a variety of cooking utensils such as spatulas, ladles, and tongs.

Preparation Techniques

In addition to having the right equipment, there are also several preparation techniques that can make meal preparation easier. These include mise en place, or having all ingredients measured and prepared before beginning to cook, and using the right cutting techniques to ensure that food is evenly cooked and aesthetically pleasing. Other techniques include using the right temperature for cooking different types of food, and knowing how to properly season dishes to enhance flavor.

Cooking For Dietary Restrictions

When cooking for individuals with dietary restrictions, such as those with food allergies or on specific diets, it is important to have a clear understanding of the restrictions and the ingredients that are allowed. This may involve substituting certain ingredients or using specific preparation techniques to ensure that the dish is safe and appropriate for the individual's needs.

CHAPTER FOUR

Following a Full Liquid Diet

Tips For Sticking To Full Liquid Diet

A full liquid diet consists of consuming only liquids or foods that turn into a liquid at room temperature. This type of diet is often prescribed for medical reasons such as preparation for a medical procedure or to ease digestive issues. However, sticking to a full liquid diet can be challenging, especially for those used to eating solid foods. Here are some tips for sticking to a full liquid diet:

1. **Plan your meals**: Planning your meals in advance can help you stick to your full liquid diet. Consult with a dietitian or healthcare professional to create a meal plan that meets your nutritional needs while sticking to the full liquid diet. Having a plan can also help you resist the temptation to eat solid foods.

2. **Experiment with different liquids**: There are a variety of liquids that can be consumed on a full liquid diet. Experimenting with different liquids can help you find options that you enjoy and can help prevent boredom. Some examples of liquids that can be consumed on a full liquid diet include broths, clear soups, milk, yogurt, smoothies, and fruit juices.

3. **Use a straw**: Using a straw can help you consume liquids more easily and can make the process of drinking more enjoyable.

4. **Blend your meals**: If you are allowed to consume blended foods, consider blending fruits or vegetables with liquids to create a nutritious and satisfying meal.

5. **Stay hydrated**: Consuming enough fluids is essential when on a full liquid diet. Drinking water or other low-calorie fluids can help you stay hydrated and feel fuller for longer periods of time.

6. **Get support**: Sticking to a full liquid diet can be challenging, especially if you are used to eating solid foods. Seek support from friends, family, or a support group to help you stay on track and motivated.

Dealing With Hunger And Cravings

Hunger and cravings are common side effects of full liquid

diets. The lack of solid food can make it challenging to feel full, and cravings can be difficult to ignore. Here are some tips for dealing with hunger and cravings when on a full liquid diet:

1. **Stay hydrated**: Consuming enough fluids can help you feel fuller for longer periods of time. Drinking water or other low-calorie fluids can also help curb cravings.

2. **Choose high-fiber liquids**: Choosing liquids that are high in fiber can help you feel full for longer periods of time. Examples of high-fiber liquids include vegetable juice and smoothies with added fiber.

3. **Try low-calorie snacks**: If you are allowed to consume snacks on your full liquid diet, consider low-calorie options such as sugar-free gelatin or pudding.

4. **Stay busy**: Distractions such as reading a book, watching a movie, or doing a hobby can help take your mind off hunger and cravings.

5. **Seek support**: Seeking support from friends, family, or a support group can help you deal with the emotional side of hunger and cravings.

Coping With The Side Effects Of Full Liquid

Diet

Full liquid diets can have side effects that can be challenging to cope with. These side effects can include nausea, constipation, and fatigue. Here are some tips for coping with the side effects of a full liquid diet:

1. **Take it slow**: Start slowly when beginning a full liquid diet to help your body adjust. Gradually increase the amount and types of liquids you consume to reduce the risk of side effects.

2. **Stay hydrated**: Drinking enough fluids is essential when on a full liquid diet. It can help prevent dehydration, which can worsen side effects.

3. **Talk to your healthcare provider**: If you are experiencing side effects that are interfering with your daily life, speak to your healthcare provider. They may be able to offer suggestions or medications to help alleviate the side effects.

4. **Consider supplements**: A full liquid diet can be low in certain nutrients, such as protein, iron, and vitamin B12. Speak to your healthcare provider or a dietitian to determine if you need to take supplements to meet your nutritional needs.

5. **Rest and conserve energy**: Fatigue can be a side effect of a full liquid diet, so it's important to

rest and conserve your energy. Avoid strenuous activities and take breaks throughout the day to help combat fatigue.

6. **Stay positive**: Staying positive and focusing on the benefits of the full liquid diet can help you cope with the side effects. Remind yourself of the medical reasons for following the diet and the positive impact it can have on your health.

How Long To Follow A Full Liquid Diet

The length of time to follow a full liquid diet can vary depending on the reason for the diet. In some cases, it may be only for a few days, while in others, it may be for several weeks. Here are some factors that may influence how long you need to follow a full liquid diet:

1. **Medical procedure**: If the full liquid diet is for a medical procedure, such as before a colonoscopy, the length of time may be only a few days.

2. **Digestive issues**: If the full liquid diet is to ease digestive issues, such as after surgery, the length of time may be several weeks.

3. **Weight loss**: If the full liquid diet is for weight loss, the length of time can vary depending on the amount of weight loss desired.

It's important to consult with a healthcare professional or a registered dietitian before starting a full liquid diet for weight loss.

4. **Overall health**: Your overall health and medical history may also influence how long you need to follow a full liquid diet. Speak to your healthcare provider to determine the appropriate length of time to follow the diet.

CHAPTER FIVE

*Health Risks Associated
with Full Liquid Diet*

Possible Nutritional Deficiencies

Nutritional deficiencies occur when the body lacks certain essential nutrients needed to function optimally. These deficiencies can have negative effects on physical and mental health. Some of the common nutritional deficiencies include:

- **Iron deficiency:** Iron is an essential mineral that plays a crucial role in the formation of red blood cells. A lack of iron in the body can lead to anemia, fatigue, weakness, and poor concentration. Iron deficiency is common among women of reproductive age and vegetarians.

- **Vitamin D deficiency:** Vitamin D is important for bone health and immune function. A lack of vitamin D in the body can lead to rickets in children and osteomalacia in adults. It can also increase the risk of autoimmune diseases, infections, and certain cancers.

- **Vitamin B12 deficiency:** Vitamin B12 is essential for nerve and brain function, as well as the production of red blood cells. A lack of vitamin B12 in the body can lead to anemia, fatigue, weakness, and numbness or tingling in the hands and feet. It is more common in vegans and elderly people.

- **Calcium deficiency:** Calcium is important for bone and teeth health, as well as muscle function and blood clotting. A lack of calcium in the body can lead to osteoporosis, muscle cramps, and heart problems.

- **Magnesium deficiency:** Magnesium is important for muscle and nerve function, as well as bone health and energy metabolism. A lack of magnesium in the body can lead to muscle cramps, fatigue, and mental health problems.

To prevent nutritional deficiencies, it is important to eat a well-balanced diet that includes a variety of fruits, vegetables, whole grains, lean proteins, and healthy fats. It may also be necessary to take supplements if you are at risk of a deficiency or have a medical condition that affects nutrient absorption.

Negative Effects On Digestive System

The digestive system is responsible for breaking down food into nutrients that the body can absorb and use for energy, growth, and repair. However, certain factors can negatively affect the digestive system and lead to various problems. Some of the negative effects on the digestive system include:

- **Poor diet:** Eating a diet high in processed foods, sugar, and unhealthy fats can disrupt the natural balance of bacteria in the gut and lead to inflammation, bloating, and constipation.

- **Stress:** Chronic stress can affect the digestive system by causing inflammation, reducing blood flow to the intestines, and altering gut bacteria.

- **Alcohol and caffeine:** Consuming too much alcohol or caffeine can irritate the lining of the stomach and intestines, leading to acid reflux, bloating, and diarrhea.

- **Medications:** Certain medications, such as antibiotics, nonsteroidal anti-inflammatory drugs (NSAIDs), and proton pump inhibitors (PPIs), can disrupt the natural balance of bacteria in the gut and cause digestive problems.

- **Medical conditions:** Medical conditions, such as inflammatory bowel disease (IBD), celiac disease, and irritable bowel syndrome (IBS), can cause chronic digestive problems and lead to malabsorption of nutrients.

To maintain a healthy digestive system, it is important to eat a balanced diet that is high in fiber, stay hydrated, manage stress, limit alcohol and caffeine intake, and talk to your healthcare provider about any medications or medical conditions that may affect your digestion.

Contraindications For Full Liquid Diet

A full liquid diet is a type of diet that includes only liquids or foods that turn into a liquid at room temperature. This type of diet is often prescribed for people who have difficulty swallowing or have had certain medical procedures. However, there are some contraindications for a full liquid diet that should be considered.

- **Malnourishment:** A full liquid diet may not provide enough essential nutrients and calories for some individuals, particularly those who are already malnourished. In such cases, a full liquid diet may worsen the condition and lead to further health problems.

- **Diabetes:** A full liquid diet that includes sugary drinks and fruit juices can cause spikes in blood sugar levels, making it unsuitable for individuals with diabetes. In such cases, a modified full liquid diet that is low in sugar and high in protein may be more appropriate.

- **Gastrointestinal problems:** A full liquid diet may not be suitable for individuals with certain gastrointestinal problems, such as diarrhea or vomiting. In such cases, a clear liquid diet may be recommended until the symptoms subside.

- **Pregnancy and breastfeeding:** Pregnant and breastfeeding women require additional nutrients and calories to support the growth and development of the fetus or infant. A full liquid diet may not provide enough of these nutrients, making it unsuitable for such individuals.

- **Allergies and intolerances:** A full liquid diet may include foods or liquids that individuals are allergic or intolerant to, which can lead to allergic reactions or digestive problems.

It is important to consult with a healthcare provider before starting a full liquid diet to ensure that it is safe and appropriate for your individual needs and medical conditions. In some cases, a modified full liquid diet or other dietary modifications may be recommended instead.

CHAPTER SIX

*Transitioning from Full Liquid
Diet to Solid Foods*

Gradual Introduction Of Solid Foods

Gradually introducing solid foods to infants is an important milestone in their development. While the American Academy of Pediatrics recommends exclusive breastfeeding for the first six months of an infant's life, introducing solid foods around six months of age is important to provide adequate nutrition and to help develop the infant's oral and motor skills.

When introducing solid foods, parents should start with small amounts of single-ingredient foods, such as rice cereal, pureed vegetables, or fruits. It is important to introduce new foods one at a time and wait a few days between introducing new foods to watch for any allergic reactions.

Here Are Some Tips For Parents When Introducing Solid Foods To Infants:

1. Start with a small amount of food and gradually increase the amount as the infant becomes more comfortable with eating.

2. Use a soft-tipped spoon and feed the infant in a semi-upright position to prevent choking.

3. Offer breast milk or formula first before introducing solid foods.

4. Introduce new foods one at a time and wait a few days between introducing new foods to watch for any allergic reactions.

5. Gradually increase the texture of the food as the infant becomes more comfortable with eating, eventually introducing mashed or chopped foods.

6. Offer a variety of foods to ensure the infant is receiving a balanced diet.

7. Avoid adding salt, sugar, or honey to the infant's food.

8. Pay attention to the infant's cues and stop

feeding when the infant shows signs of being full.

Gradual introduction of solid foods is an important milestone for infants, but it is important for parents to follow these tips to ensure the infant is receiving proper nutrition and to prevent choking or allergic reactions.

Recommended Foods For Transition

When transitioning from a liquid diet to a solid diet, it is important to introduce foods that are easy to digest and provide proper nutrition. The diet should include a variety of foods from all food groups, including fruits, vegetables, grains, proteins, and dairy.

Here Are Some Recommended Foods For Transitioning From A Liquid Diet To A Solid Diet:

1. Cooked vegetables: Soft cooked vegetables, such as sweet potatoes, carrots, and green beans, are easy to digest and provide important nutrients, including vitamin A and fiber.

2. Mashed fruits: Soft, mashed fruits, such as bananas, pears, and avocados, are easy to digest and provide important nutrients, including vitamin C and potassium.

3. Soft grains: Cooked, soft grains, such as rice or oatmeal, are easy to digest and provide important nutrients, including carbohydrates and fiber.

4. Protein-rich foods: Soft, cooked meats or legumes, such as lentils or beans, provide important nutrients, including protein and iron.

5. Dairy: Yogurt or soft cheeses, such as cottage cheese or ricotta cheese, provide important nutrients, including calcium and protein.

It is important to introduce new foods gradually and watch for any allergic reactions. Parents should also avoid adding salt, sugar, or honey to the infant's food and offer a variety of foods to ensure the infant is receiving a balanced diet.

How To Avoid Overeating After Full Liquid Diet

After a full liquid diet, it is important to gradually introduce solid foods to prevent overeating and digestive issues. The transition from a liquid diet to a solid diet should be done slowly, introducing small amounts of soft, easy-to-digest foods, and gradually increasing the amount and texture of the food.

It is also important to pay attention to the body's cues and stop eating when feeling full. Overeating after a liquid diet can cause discomfort, bloating, and other digestive issues.

Here Are Some Tips For Avoiding Overeating After A Full Liquid Diet:

1. Introduce solid foods gradually: Start with small amounts of soft, easy-to-digest foods, such as cooked vegetables or mashed fruits, and gradually increase the amount and texture of the food.

2. Pay attention to hunger cues: After a liquid diet, the stomach may not be used to solid food, so it is important to pay attention to the body's cues and stop eating when feeling full.

3. Eat slowly: Eating slowly allows the body to register when it is full, which can prevent overeating.

4. Stay hydrated: Drinking plenty of water can

help prevent overeating by filling up the stomach and reducing feelings of hunger.

5. Avoid distractions: Eating while distracted, such as watching TV or using a phone, can lead to overeating because it can be easy to lose track of how much is being eaten.

6. Chew thoroughly: Chewing thoroughly allows the body to properly digest the food, which can prevent discomfort and bloating.

7. Avoid high-fat or high-sugar foods: These types of foods can be difficult to digest and can lead to overeating.

8. Eat small, frequent meals: Eating small, frequent meals can help regulate the appetite and prevent overeating.

By following these tips, individuals can successfully transition from a full liquid diet to a solid diet without overeating or experiencing digestive issues. It is important to listen to the body's cues and take the transition slowly to ensure a successful transition.

CHAPTER SEVEN

*Frequently Asked Questions
about Full Liquid Diet*

Full Liquid Diet And Weight Loss

A Full Liquid Diet is a type of diet that is often prescribed by healthcare professionals for individuals who are unable to tolerate solid foods due to medical reasons or those recovering from surgery. The Full Liquid Diet involves consuming only liquids or foods that are liquid at room temperature for a certain period of time. These can include things like milk, juices, broths, soups, and smoothies. While a Full Liquid Diet can be effective in helping individuals lose weight, it is important to approach it with caution and under the guidance of a healthcare professional.

One of the primary ways that a Full Liquid Diet can help

with weight loss is by reducing caloric intake. Liquids tend to be lower in calories than solid foods, and so by consuming only liquids, individuals may be able to achieve a calorie deficit that can lead to weight loss. Additionally, liquids can help to promote feelings of fullness and satiety, which can help to prevent overeating and snacking on high-calorie foods.

However, it is important to note that a Full Liquid Diet can also be deficient in important nutrients and may not provide enough calories or protein for some individuals. Additionally, a Full Liquid Diet is not a sustainable long-term solution for weight loss and may lead to the loss of muscle mass rather than fat mass. Therefore, it is important to use a Full Liquid Diet as a short-term tool under the guidance of a healthcare professional.

Full Liquid Diet And Certain Illnesses

A Full Liquid Diet can be useful in the treatment of certain illnesses or conditions, such as digestive disorders or surgeries that require the avoidance of solid foods.

For example, a Full Liquid Diet may be prescribed to individuals who have had gastrointestinal surgery or who are experiencing a flare-up of Crohn's disease or ulcerative colitis.

Additionally, a Full Liquid Diet may be recommended for individuals with dysphagia or difficulty swallowing. Dysphagia can be caused by a number of underlying conditions, such as stroke, Parkinson's disease, or multiple sclerosis. A Full Liquid Diet can help to ensure that individuals with dysphagia are able to get the nutrients they need while also reducing the risk of choking or aspiration.

It is important to note, however, that a Full Liquid Diet should only be used under the guidance of a healthcare professional and should not be used as a substitute for medical treatment or medication. Additionally, a Full Liquid Diet may not be appropriate for all individuals with certain illnesses or conditions and may need to be modified or supplemented with additional nutrients.

Full Liquid Diet And Athletes

A Full Liquid Diet is not typically recommended for athletes, as it may not provide the necessary nutrients and energy needed for high-intensity physical activity. Athletes require a balance of carbohydrates, protein, and fat to fuel their workouts and promote muscle recovery and growth.

However, there may be certain circumstances where a Full Liquid Diet could be beneficial for athletes. For example, if an athlete has undergone surgery or has a digestive disorder that makes it difficult to tolerate solid foods, a Full Liquid Diet may be prescribed as a temporary measure. Additionally, some athletes may use liquid meal replacements or protein shakes as a supplement to their regular diet to promote muscle growth and recovery.

It is important for athletes to approach a Full Liquid Diet with caution and to consult with a healthcare professional or registered dietitian to ensure that they are getting the necessary nutrients and calories to support their athletic performance.

Safe Duration Of Full Liquid Diet

The length of time that an individual can safely follow a Full Liquid Diet will depend on a number of factors, including the reason for the diet and the individual's overall health status. In general, a Full Liquid Diet is not intended to be a long-term solution for weight loss or nutritional deficiencies.

If a Full Liquid Diet is being used to manage a medical condition or to aid in recovery from surgery, the length of time may be determined by the healthcare professional overseeing the individual's care. For example, if an individual has had gastrointestinal surgery, they may be instructed to follow a Full Liquid Diet for a few days before gradually transitioning back to solid foods.

If a Full Liquid Diet is being used for weight loss, it is important to approach it with caution and under the guidance of a healthcare professional or registered dietitian. A Full Liquid Diet should not be followed for an extended period of time, as it may lead to nutrient deficiencies and may not provide enough calories or protein to support overall health.

In general, a Full Liquid Diet should only be followed for

a short period of time, typically no longer than a few days to a week. Individuals who are considering a Full Liquid Diet for any reason should consult with a healthcare professional or registered dietitian to ensure that it is appropriate for their individual needs and that they are getting the necessary nutrients and calories to support their overall health.

Additionally, it is important to note that a Full Liquid Diet can be difficult to follow for an extended period of time. Liquid diets can be monotonous and may lead to feelings of deprivation and hunger, which can ultimately lead to binge eating or overeating once the diet is discontinued. It is important to have a plan in place for transitioning back to solid foods and for maintaining healthy eating habits once the Full Liquid Diet is no longer necessary.

If an individual is considering a Full Liquid Diet for weight loss, it is important to approach it with a healthy and sustainable mindset. Rather than using a Full Liquid Diet as a quick fix, individuals should focus on making long-term changes to their diet and lifestyle that can lead to sustainable weight loss and overall health improvements.

CHAPTER EIGHT

Cream of Mushroom Soup

This creamy mushroom soup is perfect for a cold day or as a starter for a dinner party. The earthy flavor of the mushrooms and the creaminess of the soup will leave you wanting more.

Ingredients:

- 1 pound mushrooms, sliced
- 1 onion, chopped
- 2 cloves garlic, minced
- 4 cups chicken or vegetable broth
- 1 cup heavy cream
- 2 tablespoons butter
- Salt and pepper, to taste
- Fresh parsley, chopped, for garnish

Instructions:

1. In a large pot, melt the butter over medium heat. Add the onions and garlic and cook until softened.

2. Add the sliced mushrooms and cook until they are soft and browned, about 10 minutes.

3. Pour in the broth and bring to a boil. Reduce heat and let simmer for 20 minutes.

4. Using an immersion blender or a regular blender, blend the soup until smooth.

5. Add the heavy cream and stir until fully incorporated. Season with salt and pepper to taste.

6. Serve hot, garnished with fresh parsley.

Nutritional Information:

- Calories: 280
- Fat: 22g
- Protein: 7g
- Carbohydrates: 15g
- Fiber: 2g

Tomato Soup

Tomato soup is a classic comfort food that is easy to make and delicious to eat. This recipe is perfect for a quick and easy lunch or dinner.

Ingredients:

- 2 tablespoons butter
- 1 onion, chopped
- 2 cloves garlic, minced
- 4 cups chicken or vegetable broth
- 2 cans (28 oz each) crushed tomatoes
- 1 teaspoon sugar
- Salt and pepper, to taste
- Fresh basil, chopped, for garnish

Instructions:

1. In a large pot, melt the butter over medium heat. Add the onions and garlic and cook until softened.

2. Add the crushed tomatoes and broth, and bring to a boil. Reduce heat and let simmer for 20 minutes.

3. Using an immersion blender or a regular blender, blend the soup until smooth.

4. Add the sugar and season with salt and pepper to taste.

5. Serve hot, garnished with fresh basil.

Nutritional Information:

- Calories: 190

- Fat: 7g
- Protein: 7g
- Carbohydrates: 25g
- Fiber: 7g

Chicken Noodle Soup (Strained)

This chicken noodle soup is perfect for those who prefer a smooth texture. The strained soup is easy on the stomach and the addition of noodles makes it a complete meal.

Ingredients:

- 1 pound boneless, skinless chicken breasts
- 4 cups chicken broth
- 2 carrots, peeled and chopped
- 2 celery stalks, chopped
- 1 onion, chopped
- 2 cloves garlic, minced
- 1 bay leaf
- Salt and pepper, to taste
- 8 oz egg noodles

Instructions:

1. In a large pot, bring the chicken broth to a boil. Add the chicken breasts, carrots, celery, onion,

garlic, bay leaf, salt, and pepper.

2. Reduce heat and let simmer for 30 minutes, or until the chicken is cooked through.

3. Remove the chicken from the pot and shred with a fork. Set aside.

4. Using a fine mesh strainer or a cheesecloth, strain the soup into a separate pot, discarding the solids.

5. Add the egg noodles to the soup and cook according to package instructions.

6. Once the noodles are cooked, add the shredded chicken to the pot and stir until heated through. 7. Serve hot.

Nutritional Information:

- Calories: 280
- Fat: 4g
- Protein: 24g
- Carbohydrates: 35g
- Fiber: 3g

Butternut Squash Soup

This creamy butternut squash soup is a perfect fall or winter dish. The sweet and savory flavors of the squash, onions, and spices make this soup a real treat.

Ingredients:

- 1 butternut squash, peeled, seeded, and cubed
- 1 onion, chopped
- 2 cloves garlic, minced
- 4 cups chicken or vegetable broth
- 1 cup heavy cream
- 2 tablespoons olive oil
- 1 teaspoon ground cinnamon
- 1/4 teaspoon ground nutmeg
- Salt and pepper, to taste
- Fresh parsley, chopped, for garnish

Instructions:

1. In a large pot, heat the olive oil over medium heat. Add the onions and garlic and cook until softened.

2. Add the cubed butternut squash, cinnamon, nutmeg, and broth. Bring to a boil, then reduce heat and let simmer for 20 minutes.

3. Using an immersion blender or a regular blender, blend the soup until smooth.

4. Add the heavy cream and stir until fully incorporated. Season with salt and pepper to taste.

5. Serve hot, garnished with fresh parsley.

Nutritional Information:

- Calories: 310
- Fat: 25g
- Protein: 5g
- Carbohydrates: 20g
- Fiber: 4g

Fish or Chicken Broth

This fish or chicken broth is perfect for those who are feeling under the weather or in need of a quick and easy meal. The simplicity of this recipe allows for the natural flavors of the fish or chicken to shine through.

Ingredients:

- 1 pound fish bones or chicken bones
- 8 cups water
- Salt and pepper, to taste

Instructions:

1. In a large pot, add the fish or chicken bones and water.

2. Bring to a boil, then reduce heat and let simmer for at least 1 hour.

3. Remove the bones from the pot using a slotted spoon or a fine mesh strainer.

4. Season with salt and pepper to taste.

5. Serve hot.

Nutritional Information:

- Calories: 0 (broth has no calories)
- Fat: 0g
- Protein: 0g
- Carbohydrates: 0g

Cream of Potato Soup

This creamy potato soup is perfect for a cold day or as a starter for a dinner party. The addition of bacon and chives makes this soup extra special.

Ingredients:

- 6 potatoes, peeled and cubed
- 1 onion, chopped
- 2 cloves garlic, minced

- 4 cups chicken or vegetable broth

- 1 cup heavy cream

- 4 slices bacon, cooked and crumbled

- 2 tablespoons butter

- Salt and pepper, to taste

- Fresh chives, chopped, for garnish

Instructions:

1. In a large pot, melt the butter over medium heat. Add the onions and garlic and cook until softened.

2. Add the cubed potatoes and broth. Bring to a boil, then reduce heat and let simmer for 20 minutes, or until the potatoes are soft.

3. Using an immersion blender or a regular blender, blend the soup until smooth.

4. Add the heavy cream and stir until fully incorporated. Season with salt and pepper to taste.

5. Serve hot, garnished with crumbled bacon and fresh chives.

Nutritional Information:

- Calories: 420

- Fat: 30g

- Protein: 8g

- Carbohydrates: 30g
- Fiber: 4g

Cream of Broccoli Soup

This cream of broccoli soup is a healthy and delicious way to enjoy this nutritious vegetable. The addition of cream and cheddar cheese gives it a rich and creamy texture.

Ingredients:

- 1 head broccoli, chopped
- 1 onion, chopped
- 2 cloves garlic, minced
- 4 cups chicken or vegetable broth
- 1 cup heavy cream
- 1 cup cheddar cheese, shredded
- 2 tablespoons butter
- Salt and pepper, to taste

Instructions:

1. In a large pot, melt the butter over medium heat. Add the onions and garlic and cook until softened.

2. Add the chopped broccoli and broth. Bring to a boil, then reduce heat and let simmer for 20 minutes, or until the broccoli is tender.

3. Using an immersion blender or a regular blender, blend the soup until smooth.

4. Add the heavy cream and shredded cheddar cheese and stir until fully incorporated. Season with salt and pepper to taste.

5. Serve hot.

Nutritional Information:

- Calories: 420
- Fat: 35g
- Protein: 10g
- Carbohydrates: 14g
- Fiber: 4g

Cream of Spinach Soup

This cream of spinach soup is a healthy and delicious way to enjoy this leafy green vegetable. The addition of cream and Parmesan cheese gives it a rich and flavorful taste.

Ingredients:

- 1 pound fresh spinach, chopped
- 1 onion, chopped
- 2 cloves garlic, minced
- 4 cups chicken or vegetable broth
- 1 cup heavy cream
- 1 cup Parmesan cheese, grated
- 2 tablespoons butter
- Salt and pepper, to taste

Instructions:

1. In a large pot, melt the butter over medium heat. Add the onions and garlic and cook until softened.

2. Add the chopped spinach and broth. Bring to a boil, then reduce heat and let simmer for 20 minutes, or until the spinach is wilted and tender.

3. Using an immersion blender or a regular blender, blend the soup until smooth.

4. Add the heavy cream and grated Parmesan cheese and stir until fully incorporated. Season with salt and pepper to taste.

5. Serve hot.

Nutritional Information:

- Calories: 390
- Fat: 30g
- Protein: 18g
- Carbohydrates: 12g
- Fiber: 4g

Miso Soup

This classic Japanese soup is made with miso paste, which gives it a salty and savory flavor. The addition of tofu and seaweed makes it a hearty and healthy meal.

Ingredients:

- 4 cups water
- 4 tablespoons miso paste
- 1 block tofu, cubed
- 1/4 cup seaweed, chopped
- 2 green onions, sliced
- 1 teaspoon sesame oil

Instructions:

1. In a large pot, bring the water to a boil.

2. Reduce heat and add the miso paste, stirring until fully dissolved.

3. Add the cubed tofu and chopped seaweed and let simmer for 5 minutes.

4. Remove from heat and add the sliced green onions and sesame oil.

5. Serve hot.

Nutritional Information:

- Calories: 160
- Fat: 8g
- Protein: 13g
- Carbohydrates: 13g
- Fiber: 2g

Vegetable Soup (Strained)

This vegetable soup is a simple and healthy way to get your daily dose of veggies. Straining the soup gives it a smooth and creamy texture, while keeping it low in calories and fat.

Ingredients:

- 2 carrots, chopped
- 2 celery stalks, chopped
- 1 onion, chopped
- 2 cloves garlic, minced
- 4 cups chicken or vegetable broth
- Salt and pepper, to taste

Instructions:

1. In a large pot, sauté the onions and garlic over medium heat until softened.

2. Add the chopped carrots, celery, and broth. Bring to a boil, then reduce heat and let simmer for 20 minutes, or until the vegetables are tender.

3. Using an immersion blender or a regular blender, blend the soup until smooth.

4. Strain the soup through a fine-mesh sieve to remove any chunks or fibers.

5. Season with salt and pepper to taste.

6. Serve hot.

Nutritional Information:

- Calories: 70
- Fat: 1g
- Protein: 2g

- Carbohydrates: 14g
- Fiber: 3g

Fruit Smoothie (with Yogurt or Milk)

This fruit smoothie is a healthy and refreshing way to start your day. The addition of yogurt or milk gives it a creamy and satisfying texture.

Ingredients:

- 1 banana, sliced
- 1 cup strawberries, sliced
- 1/2 cup plain yogurt or milk
- 1 tablespoon honey

Instructions:

1. In a blender, combine the sliced banana, sliced strawberries, yogurt or milk, and honey.

2. Blend on high speed until smooth and creamy.

3. Pour into a glass and serve cold.

Nutritional Information:

- Calories: 190
- Fat: 2g
- Protein: 6g

- Carbohydrates: 41g
- Fiber: 4g

Protein Shake

This protein shake is a great way to refuel your body after a workout. The addition of protein powder and almond milk gives it a creamy and satisfying texture.

Ingredients:

- 1 scoop vanilla protein powder
- 1 cup unsweetened almond milk
- 1/2 banana, sliced
- 1/2 cup ice cubes

Instructions:

1. In a blender, combine the protein powder, almond milk, sliced banana, and ice cubes.

2. Blend on high speed until smooth and creamy.

3. Pour into a glass and serve cold.

Nutritional Information:

- Calories: 210

- Fat: 4g
- Protein: 25g
- Carbohydrates: 19g
- Fiber: 4g

Hot Chocolate (Made with Milk)

This hot chocolate is a classic and comforting drink that is perfect for a cold winter day. The use of milk instead of water gives it a rich and creamy texture.

Ingredients:

- 2 cups milk
- 1/4 cup unsweetened cocoa powder
- 1/4 cup sugar
- 1 teaspoon vanilla extract

Instructions:

1. In a medium saucepan, heat the milk over medium-low heat until hot but not boiling.

2. Whisk in the cocoa powder, sugar, and vanilla extract until fully incorporated.

3. Continue to heat and whisk until the mixture is smooth and creamy.

4. Pour into mugs and serve hot.

Nutritional Information:

- Calories: 220
- Fat: 6g
- Protein: 8g
- Carbohydrates: 34g
- Fiber

Fruit Juice (Strained)

This fruit juice is a refreshing and healthy way to get your daily dose of vitamins and minerals. Straining the juice removes any pulp or fibers, giving it a smooth and easy-to-drink texture.

Ingredients:

- 2 apples, cored and chopped
- 2 oranges, peeled and segmented
- 1 cup grapes
- 1/2 lemon, juiced

Instructions:

1. In a juicer, combine the chopped apples, segmented oranges, grapes, and lemon juice.

2. Juice the ingredients until fully extracted.

3. Strain the juice through a fine-mesh sieve to remove any pulp or fibers.

4. Serve the juice cold.

Nutritional Information:

- Calories: 150
- Fat: 1g
- Protein: 2g
- Carbohydrates: 38g
- Fiber: 3g

Vegetable Juice (Strained)

This vegetable juice is a healthy and refreshing way to get your daily dose of veggies. Straining the juice removes any pulp or fibers, giving it a smooth and easy-to-drink texture.

Ingredients:

- 2 carrots, chopped
- 2 celery stalks, chopped
- 1 beet, chopped
- 1/2 lemon, juiced

Instructions:

1. In a juicer, combine the chopped carrots, chopped celery, chopped beet, and lemon juice.

2. Juice the ingredients until fully extracted.

3. Strain the juice through a fine-mesh sieve to remove any pulp or fibers.

4. Serve the juice cold.

Nutritional Information:

- Calories: 70
- Fat: 0g
- Protein: 2g
- Carbohydrates: 16g
- Fiber: 4g

Tomato Juice (Strained)

This tomato juice is a classic and refreshing drink that is perfect for any time of day. Straining the juice removes any seeds or fibers, giving it a smooth and easy-to-drink texture.

Ingredients:

- 4 tomatoes, chopped
- 1/2 lemon, juiced
- Salt and pepper, to taste

Instructions:

1. In a juicer, combine the chopped tomatoes and lemon juice.
2. Juice the ingredients until fully extracted.
3. Strain the juice through a fine-mesh sieve to remove any seeds or fibers.
4. Season with salt and pepper to taste.
5. Serve the juice cold.

Nutritional Information:

- Calories: 50
- Fat: 0g
- Protein: 2g
- Carbohydrates: 12g
- Fiber: 3g

Vanilla or Chocolate Pudding

This pudding is a classic and comforting dessert that is sure to satisfy your sweet tooth. The addition of vanilla or chocolate gives it a rich and indulgent flavor.

Ingredients:

- 1/2 cup sugar
- 1/4 cup cornstarch
- 1/4 teaspoon salt
- 2 cups milk
- 2 egg yolks
- 2 tablespoons unsalted butter
- 1 teaspoon vanilla extract or 1/4 cup unsweetened cocoa powder (for chocolate pudding)

Instructions:

1. In a medium saucepan, whisk together the sugar, cornstarch, and salt.
2. Slowly whisk in the milk until fully incorporated.
3. Whisk in the egg yolks and butter until fully incorporated.
4. Cook over medium heat, stirring constantly, until the mixture thickens and comes to a boil.
5. Reduce heat and continue to cook for 2-3

minutes, stirring constantly, until the mixture is thick and smooth.

7. Remove from heat and stir in the vanilla extract or cocoa powder (for chocolate pudding) until fully incorporated.

8. Pour the mixture into individual serving dishes.

9. Cover with plastic wrap and refrigerate for at least 2 hours, or until set.

10. Serve chilled.

Nutritional Information:

- Vanilla Pudding:
    - Calories: 200
    - Fat: 6g
    - Protein: 4g
    - Carbohydrates: 34g
    - Fiber: 0g
- Chocolate Pudding:
    - Calories: 230
    - Fat: 8g
    - Protein: 5g
    - Carbohydrates: 37g
    - Fiber: 2g

Custard

This classic dessert is a creamy and delicious way to end any meal. The addition of vanilla gives it a warm and comforting flavor.

Ingredients:

- 2 cups milk
- 4 egg yolks
- 1/4 cup sugar
- 1 teaspoon vanilla extract

Instructions:

1. Preheat the oven to 325°F (165°C).

2. In a medium saucepan, heat the milk over medium heat until it just begins to simmer.

3. In a separate mixing bowl, whisk together the egg yolks and sugar until light and fluffy.

4. Slowly whisk in the hot milk, stirring constantly.

5. Stir in the vanilla extract.

6. Pour the mixture into 4-6 individual ramekins.

7. Place the ramekins in a baking dish and pour hot water into the dish until it reaches halfway up the sides of the ramekins.

8. Bake for 35-40 minutes, or until the custard is set but still slightly jiggly in the center.

9. Remove the ramekins from the water bath and let cool to room temperature.

10. Cover with plastic wrap and refrigerate for at least 2 hours, or until chilled.

11. Serve chilled.

Nutritional Information:

- Calories: 170
- Fat: 7g
- Protein: 6g
- Carbohydrates: 20g
- Fiber: 0g

Jello or Other Gelatin Dessert

This jello or gelatin dessert is a fun and easy way to enjoy a sweet treat. The addition of fruit gives it a fresh and fruity flavor.

Ingredients:

- 1 package (3 oz) fruit-flavored gelatin

- 1 cup boiling water

- 1 cup cold water

- 1 cup fresh fruit (such as sliced strawberries or blueberries)

Instructions:

1. In a mixing bowl, dissolve the gelatin in boiling water.

2. Stir in the cold water and fresh fruit.

3. Pour the mixture into a mold or individual serving dishes.

4. Refrigerate for 2-3 hours, or until set.

5. Serve chilled.

Nutritional Information:

- Calories: 90

- Fat: 0g

- Protein: 3g

- Carbohydrates: 22g

- Fiber: 0g

Milk-Based Ice Cream or Sorbet

This milk-based ice cream or sorbet is a creamy and refreshing treat that is perfect for any occasion. The addition of fresh fruit gives it a sweet and fruity flavor.

Ingredients:

- 2 cups whole milk
- 1 cup heavy cream
- 3/4 cup sugar
- 2 teaspoons vanilla extract or 2 cups fresh fruit
- 1/4 teaspoon salt

Instructions:

1. In a medium saucepan, combine the whole milk, heavy cream, sugar, and salt.

2. Heat the mixture over medium heat, stirring constantly, until the sugar has fully dissolved and the mixture is hot but not boiling.

3. Remove from heat and stir in the vanilla extract (if making vanilla ice cream) or the fresh fruit (if making fruit sorbet).

4. Let the mixture cool to room temperature.

5. Pour the mixture into an ice cream maker and churn according to manufacturer's instructions.

6. Transfer the ice cream or sorbet to a freezer-safe container and freeze for at least 2 hours, or until firm.

7. Serve chilled.

Nutritional Information:

- Vanilla Ice Cream:
    - Calories: 270
    - Fat: 16g
    - Protein: 4g
    - Carbohydrates: 28g
    - Fiber: 0g
- Fruit Sorbet:
    - Calories: 170
    - Fat: 3g
    - Protein: 1g
    - Carbohydrates: 37g
    - Fiber: 1g

CONCLUSION

Final Thoughts on Full Liquid Diet

A full liquid diet is a type of diet that allows for consumption of foods that are in liquid form or can be converted to liquid. It is typically used for a short period of time, such as before or after surgery, to ease digestion or manage certain medical conditions. Although it can provide some benefits, there are also some concerns and considerations that need to be taken into account. Here are some final thoughts on full liquid diet:

First and foremost, it is important to note that a full liquid diet should not be followed for an extended period of time, as it can result in nutrient deficiencies and other health problems. A full liquid diet lacks fiber, which is essential for maintaining digestive health and preventing constipation. It is also low in protein, which is necessary for building and repairing tissues, as well as maintaining a strong immune system. Therefore, it is crucial to follow a full liquid diet only for the recommended period of time and under the supervision of a healthcare provider.

Another consideration when it comes to full liquid diet is the risk of overconsumption of sugar. Many liquid foods, such as juices and smoothies, can be high in sugar, which can lead to spikes in blood sugar levels and insulin resistance over time. It is important to choose liquid foods that are low in sugar and high in nutrients, such as protein shakes and vegetable soups.

It is also important to note that a full liquid diet may not be suitable for everyone. For example, people with certain medical conditions, such as kidney disease, may need to limit their intake of certain nutrients, such as potassium and phosphorus, which can be found in some liquid foods. Additionally, people with certain allergies or intolerances may need to avoid certain liquid foods, such as dairy or soy-based products.

Finally, it is crucial to consult with a healthcare provider and a registered dietitian before starting a full liquid diet. They can help assess your individual needs and provide guidance on which liquid foods are safe and appropriate for you. They can also monitor your progress and adjust your diet as needed to ensure that you are getting the nutrients you need to maintain good health.

In conclusion, a full liquid diet can be a useful tool for managing certain medical conditions or for easing digestion before or after surgery. However, it should only be followed for a short period of time, and under the supervision of a healthcare provider. It is important to choose liquid foods that are low in sugar and high in nutrients, and to consult with a healthcare provider and a registered dietitian before starting a full liquid diet to ensure that it is safe and appropriate for you.

Importance Of Consulting A Doctor And Registered Dietitian

Consulting with a doctor and a registered dietitian is essential for maintaining good health and preventing or managing certain medical conditions. Both healthcare professionals play an important role in providing personalized care and guidance that is tailored to an individual's unique needs and goals. Here are some reasons why consulting with a doctor and a registered dietitian is so important:

First and foremost, a doctor can provide a comprehensive assessment of your health status and medical history, which can help identify any underlying health issues or risk factors that may require treatment or management. For example, a doctor can perform a physical examination, order lab tests, and review your medical records to assess your overall health and any potential health risks.

A registered dietitian, on the other hand, can provide guidance on nutrition and dietary habits that can help prevent or manage certain medical conditions. They can help you develop a healthy eating plan that is tailored to your individual needs and preferences, and can provide education on proper portion sizes, nutrient balance, and meal planning strategies. They can also provide guidance on dietary modifications that may be necessary for managing specific medical conditions, such as diabetes, high blood pressure, or kidney disease

Additionally, consulting with a registered dietitian can be particularly important for those with special dietary needs or restrictions, such as those with food allergies, intolerances, or dietary restrictions due to religious or cultural beliefs. A registered dietitian can help you navigate these challenges and provide guidance on how to ensure that your diet is still well-balanced and nutritious.

Another important reason to consult with a doctor and a registered dietitian is to help prevent and manage chronic diseases. Chronic diseases such as heart disease, diabetes, and cancer are among the leading causes of death worldwide. Many of these diseases can be prevented or managed through lifestyle modifications, such as diet and exercise. A doctor and registered dietitian can work together to develop a personalized plan to help prevent or manage chronic diseases.

Finally, consulting with a doctor and a registered dietitian can be an important step in promoting overall health and well-being. They can provide guidance on lifestyle factors such as stress management, sleep habits, and physical activity, which can all contribute to a healthy and balanced lifestyle. They can also provide support and resources for managing mental health conditions such as depression and anxiety, which can have a significant impact on overall health and well-being.

In conclusion, consulting with a doctor and a registered dietitian is essential for maintaining good health, preventing and managing chronic diseases, and promoting overall well-being. They can provide personalized care and guidance that is tailored to an individual's unique needs and goals, and can help ensure that you are getting the nutrients and care you need to lead a healthy and fulfilling life. If you have any questions or concerns about your health or diet, consider scheduling an appointment with a healthcare provider and a registered dietitian to discuss your options and develop a plan that is right for you.

* 9 7 9 8 3 8 8 2 3 9 3 0 3 *